skinny jeans
...at last!

skinny jeans ...at last!

secrets to long-term weight loss surgery success

Clifton Thomas, MD

*This book is dedicated to
the many patients that inspire me*

CONTENTS

ACKNOWLEDGMENTS

Eben Pagan for his unique ability to teach many of the concepts laced throughout this book. Joseph Campbell for his unique understanding of truth as told through the stories of time. Brian Tracey for his many years of teaching concepts that empower us all. David Deida for teaching me the spiritual nature of giving your gift to the world. My parents loving influence and my uncle Clyde Thomas, M.D. for sharing with me his passion as a doctor.

Skinny Jeans....At Last

INTRODUCTION

The joy of communication comes in many forms. This book is a byproduct of my many years of talking to patients, discovering what drives a patient to seek surgery, and how the weight loss positively impacts their lives. The process of writing this book has not only been a reawakening for me, but a reminder that I am very lucky to wake up every day of my life to a profession I love, one that allows me to help people improve their own lives. I am thankful for the experiences I have had with my patients. My hope is that you will find this book inspiring, and in turn use that inspiration to live your best life possible.

With this book, I began by trying to think of who would read it and why. That's where the magic began to unfold. Although I felt I knew the answers from years of talking to patients, I starting asking specific questions. I would ask, "What was it that finally drove you to decide on surgery? Now that you have lost weight what is the specific thing you notice is better?"

What thrilled me the most was the body language and enthusiasm patients exhibited while explaining what that thing was. The magic was in the specifics of their explanations. "Well, I feel better in every way" was a common response but abstract and difficult to visualize. Then I would push for specific examples. They would begin by telling me things like, "I can finally fit into my skinny jeans."

Have you ever seen one of those rapid-sequence films of a flower blooming where the flower goes from a seedling to flower within seconds? That is what it is like to ask that question and see the emotions blossom.

I realized how powerful those emotions were and that by tapping into those emotions and getting a true feeling embedded in our memories, we could use this as a tool to overcome the nasty problem of resistance to doing what is required for long-term success.

Doctors like to focus on specific health benefits, like the fact that with surgery most patients resolve their diabetes, hypertension, hyperlipidemia, and sleep apnea. These issues are huge in the overall scheme of major medical developments. But from the patients' perspective, they are thrilled to get rid of bottles and bottles of medicine, and to be able to run or play with their children without having to quit due to shortness of breath or unbearable knee pain.

I feel that tapping into those emotions opens the door to long-term weight loss success. My hope is that you will connect with these patients' stories, that their experiences will inspire you to open that door to the secret of why success is both elusive and obvious.

Yes, you can do it too!

1
IT'S ELUSIVE
AND
THAT'S WHY IT'S A SECRET

Fitting into those skinny jeans is just a metaphor
for what it feels like to lose excess weight.
-Clifton Thomas, MD

I love the words *Elusive Obvious*. They make up the title of a book written many years ago by Moshe Feldenkrais. The book contains a lot of wisdom regarding body movement and awareness.

When something in our lives is elusive, it's like we are chasing something that we just can't seem to catch. It's always just out of reach. Weight loss advice is everywhere, so why does the ability to lose weight remain so elusive? Well, it's obvious.

Weight loss, or better yet, the mechanisms that regulate weight, is a very complex physiologic process that we are just scratching the surface of understanding.

Our bodies contain an enormous number of chemical messengers, such as hormones, which work on a method of bio-feedback and actively prevent you from losing weight. I won't bore you by listing them, but it is a fact that they exist. I think evolutionary theory explains why these chemicals exist. They were built into us for a time that no longer exists, when survival was difficult and most dependent on our ability to find food and eat. We now live in a time of food abundance.

It's also a fact that the more we learn, the less we know. Every time we identify a new chemical that may help us lose weight, there is another chemical lurking in the shadows that keeps it from happening. The bottom line is simply this, the more we learn, the more we become aware of the complexity of this weight-regulating system, and the further we seem to be from finding a magic pill.

> **Think of it as a board game that is impossible to beat but lures us into believing we can win, so we keep playing.**

Intuitively, it makes sense that if eating a lot causes us to gain weight, then starving ourselves would cause us to lose weight. It does, short term. We have all tried it, and we all know it does not work. Almost always we regain all we lost plus a ten percent gain. To beat the board game, we need to think counter intuitively.

It's obvious that we are dealing with a very complex and difficult-to-understand system, a system that seems to be beating us despite all the volumes of weight loss advice. We only know a fraction of the reasons why weight loss surgery normalizes our metabolism, but we know that it does.

There is no published medical paper on non-surgical weight loss anywhere in the world where a significant group of patients followed some method and were able to keep fifty or more pounds off for five years or longer. Zero! That tells you something. Medical doctors produce tons and tons of papers. Zero is an obviously amazing number.

The success rate of the number of people who have tried to lose fifty or more pounds and keep it off for five years is near zero. It is well documented that many methods of weight loss can help a person lose ten percent of their excess weight and keep it off for five years. Ten percent of excess weight loss does make a person much healthier, but let's put that into perspective. If you need to lose one hundred pounds, ten percent would be ten pounds. And that is not enough to fit into those skinny jeans. And please remember fitting into those skinny jeans is just a metaphor for what it feels like to lose excess weight.

The chemical changes that normalize metabolism gradually disappear over time, generally years. I think it takes one to two years to establish a habit. Long term weight loss success requires you to lock in some simple, do able eating habits. These habits work. This chemical phase, where the operation is doing the majority of the work for you, is the time to lock in these habits. If you lose focus and get lazy, you will regain weight.

We are constantly chasing new methods, expecting them to be the magic answer, yet weight loss surgery is the only proven tool for patients to lose more than ten percent of excess weight long-term. Surgery tricks this complex bio-feedback system in the body, and that's the magic of why it works. There is no magic pill that can do that, and starving does not work.

Awareness is the key to all change.

Skinny Jeans....At Last

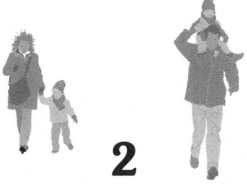

2
WHAT IT'S LIKE TO FIT INTO THOSE SKINNY JEANS

and why knowing this is the secret to all the secrets

What does fitting into those skinny jeans really mean? It goes way beyond the obvious. Being able to wear clothes that you've always fantasized about but couldn't imagine is a fabulous benefit, but it goes much further than this.

Imagine for a moment what it would feel like:

- Play with your kids or grandkids without getting short of breath.
- Get rid of bottles of medicine that treat high blood pressure, high cholesterol, and diabetes.
- Become fertile and be able to get pregnant and have children.
- Buy fashionable clothes off the rack.
- Wake up rested and full of energy because your sleep apnea has disappeared.
- See your kids or grandkids grow up with added years to your life.
- Be able to easily bend over and put your shoes on.
- Be able to buckle your seatbelt comfortably.
- Enjoy your sense of job security with renewed vigor...

We all sometimes talk in the abstract. "I just feel better." But to really know what it's like to fit into those skinny jeans we need to capture and embrace the emotion that goes along with it using very specific words of exactly *what* is better. That's when the magic occurs.

I ask patients, "Now that you have lost weight, *what* is better?" They all start off with something abstract like, "Well, I just feel better." That's when I push for specifics. These are those stories - the stories that have moved me, the stories that inspired this book, the stories about the changes in peoples' lives after losing the weight.

A buddy of mine had a lap band, and the result was that he no longer suffered from sleep apnea. I asked him *the question.*

"I'll tell you what it's like...
It's like waking up feeling ten years younger!"

Carol has been very successful with her lap band. She is a little OCD (obsessive compulsive disorder) and following rules is easy for her. I asked her *the question.* As usual, her answer was, "I just feel better." Then I pushed. Suddenly her lips widened and turned up in a smile, her face developed a glow, and her voice became louder and full of inflection.

"I can cross my legs for the first time!"

I get lots of stories about being able to buy fashionable clothes off the rack. Linda decided to have surgery because of unbearable knee pain, hypertension, and sleep apnea. But when I asked her *the question,* her voice softened and her eyes began to have that look that she was looking inside and revisiting and feeling the emotion. Enthusiastically, she said:

"I went to Victoria's Secret
and was able to buy a bra off the rack."

Terri is a thirty-five-year-old mother, wife, and nurse. Before surgery she carried herself with the posture of someone who felt good about herself.

And even though she did not have as much weight to lose as most, her weight was bothering her. She is self-motivated and has will-power, but she had tried every diet imaginable and could not lose the weight.

She had family members with much more severe weight problems and was scared of getting bigger. When I asked her *the question,* she leaned forward, her eyes soft but intense, and she answered me.

"My sex life is better!"

Terri went on to say that she and her husband love each other very much, and he never said anything or did anything for her to think otherwise. She explained, "I felt better about the way I looked. I had more energy and enthusiasm, and it showed in the bedroom." I could visualize a big smile on her husband's face.

She continued to beam, and the intensity she radiated completely filled the room. I, too, could feel that energy.

It was like she was a teenager again.

David is a good-hearted man: a husband, father, and home builder. His faith is very important to him, and you can sense how that guides his heart. His weight was causing unbearable knee pain, and his high blood pressure was getting worse.

He intuitively knew that it did not make sense to have knee surgery, that what he needed was to get all that weight off those knees. So he decided to have surgery and has been very successful maintaining an excellent weight.

His hypertension and unbearable knee pain were resolved. So when I pushed him with *the question,* he began talking about his boys. His boys play baseball. They not only play it, they live and breathe it. He talked with pride about now being their coach, no longer sitting in the stands or on the fence: he is participating. His answer to *the question* was heartwarming.

"I can finally be the father that in my heart was there. I am no longer held back by pain and shortness of breath."

Christine and her husband had been married for ten years. They both came from big families and having children and being parents was important to both of them. There was no doubt that they loved each other very much. But they had been unable to get pregnant. Christine had some hormonal issues that her gynecologist was working on but without success.

On the first office visit, the tension the situation was causing Christine was obvious. She decided to have a sleeve gastrectomy and lost her excess weight. Two years later she walked into the office carrying a car seat with her newborn baby girl, Cari. I asked her *the question* with a smile knowing quite well how she would answer.

"I get to be a mother."

It is one of those little-known secrets that when women lose significant weight, they become very fertile. Every year, some patient walks into the office carrying her newborn daughter, along with her twenty-something-year-old daughter. After many years without using contraception and not getting pregnant, and now in their forties, these patients don't believe it can happen. But it does. At first they are in shock, but then they feel reborn themselves.

Mike is an audio sound specialist. He came to the office weighing 350 pounds. He has many jobs, but one is traveling with a promotional speaker. He used to have a moment of fear as he entered a plane. He was uncertain of how the seat belt would or would not buckle, and how the person sitting beside him would respond.

Carrying luggage was a chore. He would easily get short of breath and have to stop and rest. He was too proud to ride a cart. He had a lot of equipment to set up, and that was a challenge.

He had difficulty staying awake during the talks because his sleep apnea was bad, and he rarely had a good night's sleep. He would listen to the self-help talks and ask himself *why? Why can't I have what it takes to lose weight? What's wrong with me?*

Mike had a gastric bypass and has lost his excess weight and resolved his sleep apnea.

When I asked Mike *the question,* he started like most in the abstract: "I just feel better. My health is better." I pushed and he elaborated.

"I can get on a plane and easily buckle my seat belt."

You know that look someone has when a big problem in their life has been resolved, that sense of relief that some obstacle is out of the way and now they can move forward? Mike had that look. He then went on to talk about his job and explained that he now has better job security.

Mary's kids are all grown. She is financially secure, and likes to travel. She had a gastric bypass and lost close to one hundred pounds. She stopped needing insulin for her diabetes the night of surgery. She no longer takes high blood pressure medicine, Lasix, medicine for cholesterol, acid reflux medicine, or antidepressants. Instead, she takes B12 under her tongue, a multi-vitamin, and calcium.

When I asked Mary *the question*, she responded like all the rest, "I'm healthy and I feel better." So I pushed. Then she said with excitement,

"I no longer have to lug bottles and bottles of medicine with me. The pills I now take remind me that I am healthy and trying to stay that way. Before, all those bottles reminded me I was sick and getting sicker."

She went on to describe (much like Mike) how it was so much easier to travel and to really enjoy herself.

Andrea is a relatively new mother. She has a three-year-old girl that just learned to ride a tricycle. When I asked her *the question*, she answered as abstractly as others. Then it happened.

She told me of a recent event where her daughter was riding her tricycle in the driveway. It was a beautiful spring day and everything seemed alive: the birds, the trees, and her daughter.

Suddenly her daughter raced her tricycle into the street. Out of the corner of her eye, Andrea could see a car rapidly approaching and the driver seemed mindless while talking on her cell-phone.

Andrea sprung into action and saved her daughter from being hit by the car. She said, from a deep place in her heart,

"That moment was very special to me, I was able to protect my daughter, knowing quite well that before surgery I would have been incapable of that feat."

Breaking chairs happens when you are very over weight. Jessica told me that she is more outgoing and goes more places. Before weight loss she felt like people looked and watched her differently. When I asked her *the question* and pushed for specifics, she told me,

"I was able to go to a cookout and sit in a lounge chair with no worry it was going to break. And I did not feel like people were watching me as I sat down. And I noticed that not only did I not break the chair, there was room left over. It really felt good."

****

Chemical Changes

Feeling emotion is a chemical event in our bodies, and an emotional experience is very hard to forget. So what is going on when patients regain weight after surgery? We get lazy and we forget where we were.

With the gastric bypass and the sleeve gastrectomy, there are chemical changes that stabilize the way your body handles food. In the beginning these operations do most of the work for you. This is the easiest time ever to establish good eating habits. It is easy and very doable.

> **It takes one to two years to establish a habit to the point that it becomes part of who you are.**

We are all resistant to change. Giving up the resistance to change your eating habits is the obstacle preventing you from reaching your goal of long-term weight loss success. How do you give up resistance? You tap into the emotions of that *specific thing* or *things* are that made you feel better, and feel them.

Whether it's fitting into skinny jeans or buckling your seatbelt, remember them; close your eyes and feel them deeply. Feel the way your body feels as you remember. Relive it over and over. What you will find is that there is less resistance to doing what is needed for long-term success.

Skinny Jeans....At Last

3
YOU CAN DO IT!
but why most people don't

Leslie is a mother of two boys, 6 and 8 years of age. She came to my office to learn more about the sleeve gastrectomy. Not long into the conversation she began crying and saying that she was sorry that she did not have the will power to lose the weight on her own but had to do something. She said she had tried very hard with every diet imaginable, but she just could not do it. She did not have the energy to be a good mother and was worried about her health, and possibly not surviving to see her boys grow up.

I watched as she blamed herself over and over. It was like she had been defeated, and in defeat would have to have an operation. I began talking to her about blame and how it works against her. I emphasized that nearly zero people walking in her shoes can accomplish her goal without help. We talked about how this is not a character weakness but something much more complex.

A simple observation of people she knows or has heard about who have struggled to lose weight, should tell her it is *nearly impossible* to do on her own; otherwise, more people would be successful. It is intuitively obvious. This feeling of blame, and the belief that they should be able to do it on their own, is the essence of why we only perform weight loss surgery on one percent of those who would benefit, despite overwhelming evidence that it works.

I hear patients blame themselves as they are trying to learn healthy eating habits. The energy in our bodies is much like money. We *can* control where we spend it. We *can* control whether we spend it on something of value or not. Spending our energy on blame wastes energy on something that does not help us. We need to focus on what we can control and use the tools such as impersonal techniques to learn new eating habits and giving up old habits. After weight loss surgery these are very do-able.

Most people trying to lose weight spend their energy chasing new magic methods of weight loss and blaming themselves for not having the character or will power to do it. And neither practice gives us anything of value. This is the essence of why most people cannot lose weight. They are spending their energy on something that does not work.

I want to talk about tools. Tools have great value when trying to accomplish a task (like learning new eating habits and giving up old ones, which is very doable after weight loss surgery). Just sit back and close your eyes for a moment, and walk through your day thinking of all the tools you use and how difficult life would be without them. Don't forget about that early morning cup of coffee and that early morning trip to the toilet. Every aspect of our lives uses tools to get a job done.

I like the metaphor that weight loss surgery is a tool. Tools are impersonal. Hopefully your surgeon is personable, but the actual technique of surgery is impersonal, much like working on a machine. And the biochemical pathways are impersonal much like baking bread where the right ingredients and right temperature at the right time is needed for the bread to rise.

> **Objectifying your demons robs them of the power to control you.**

Weight loss surgery and the successful habits involved in the eating rules are tools to help you lose excess weight. We are the same in that we all need tools to accomplish a complex task like losing excess weight. However, we are all different enough that we need to figure out which surgery is best for you, and tailor the eating rules and health habits so they fit *your* life.

The failures following weight loss surgery are small in number - but real. We need a shovel to dig a hole, and most can do it, but some people can't dig a hole even in sand with a tool like a shovel.

The secret to long-term weight loss surgery success begins with tapping into the strong emotions and feelings of what life is like after losing weight. Using those emotions as a key to open the door to basic changes in our day-to-day eating is instrumental for our success. The result is getting rid of that nasty thing called resistance, allowing us to accomplish something that is simple - that we know is right for us - and very doable.

If I told patients they would be given a million dollars to follow some of these eating rules, they would think it was the easiest million possible. But in contrast to losing the weight without weight loss surgery as a tool, it would be nearly impossible in the long term. Learning healthy eating habits is very doable. Losing fifty or more pounds and keeping it off long term without weight loss surgery is not.

By the way, Leslie did have a sleeve gastrectomy and lost her excess weight. Now she says, "Why did I wait so long!"

Our lives are like a movie where we get to write the script.

Skinny Jeans....At Last

4
SECRETS TO SUCCESS

These secrets are few in number and easy to understand. It is important to focus on these rules and their simplicity will help you focus. They are challenging for all of us. Our resistance to change will be the main obstacle to our success. If you give up the resistance, you will find them easy. However, giving up the resistance is not easy. Our eating habits did not develop overnight and will not resolve overnight.

You will need to develop the correct mindset to embrace your resistance and chip away at learning these rules. *This is the first and most important step toward fitting into those skinny jeans.* Learning the nutritional value of food is important, but put all your focus and energy here *first.*

Think back to a recent outing, event, vacation, family crisis or just a busy week. We live in a time with events after events after events. We all have them. Most likely, if you had spent months developing the mindset to follow these rules, perhaps one or all of these events would have sabotaged your plan to eat better. This is not a good time to beat yourself up. It is a time to look back and ask yourself: *What could I have done differently? What impersonal tool or technique could I use to help myself follow eating rules in any of these situations?* Set yourself up for success next time. And if it was unavoidable, and sometimes it is, then celebrate your understanding of the importance of these rules and focus on getting back on track.

Plan your meals and follow your plan

I have been a certified scuba diver since 1972. One of the key concepts is to *plan your dive and dive your plan.* In scuba diving it saves lives. *But* it also applies to long-term weight loss surgery success.

By following success habits and doing what it takes to fit into those skinny jeans - it may save your life as well.

I ask patients, "Are you a good planner, maybe even a little obsessive about planning?" It's fun to watch their body language. Usually the patient, (and sometimes the friend or family member) will start nodding their head up and down in agreement. Patients who plan easily, in general, do very well with long-term success.

Most of us have good intentions when planning our day, but we act haphazardly. We live in a very busy time, but we need to go to bed at night knowing exactly when and what we are going to eat the next day. Set your cell phone alarm to go off when it is a planned eating time and eat - hungry or not. Do it just like it was taking an important pill. Adjust those eating times for the next day if needed. The most important part is planning your meals and *following* your plan.

Go no more than four hours without eating
a planned meal or snack

Most people need a small meal mid-morning, mid-afternoon, or both. It all depends on when you get up, when you can schedule lunch, when you can schedule dinner, and when you go to bed. I have many patientswho are school teachers and often their scheduled lunch is at 10:30a.m. Their family eats around 7:00 p.m. They definitely need something mid-afternoon, even if it's just something like half of a protein bar or half of a banana with peanut butter. Otherwise, they will be too hungry throughout the day.

You should go no more than four hours without eating. Once you have gotten to the point of being *crazy starving hungry* you have already messed up.

It is then time to learn from your mistake and plan better for tomorrow. It is not a time to blame yourself for being weak, but a time to learn from your mistake and take action tomorrow. Chip away at it and eventually it will become what you do, a habit that you don't even need to think about.

No unplanned eating

We have to eliminate unplanned eating for long-term success. *No unplanned eating. No unplanned eating.* No unplanned eating has to be the mindset to eliminate this sneaky habit. I call "snacking" unplanned eating. It's the *see food eat food diet.*

You should not let food touch your fingers unless it is a scheduled meal time. You may have three, four, or five scheduled meal times; all are OK depending on your lifestyle at the time.

It seems counter intuitive. What is the difference between eating several things unplanned through the day and planning several times to eat? It is a mindset much like the day-to-day spending of pennies on things of little or no value. They add up and cost us dearly.

We have to eliminate unplanned eating for long-term success.

No liquid calories

If you can put something with calories in your hand that will eventually flow out of your hand, then it is in the physical state of a liquid. Liquid calories sneak up on us. Examples of liquid calories are soup, milk, orange juice, sweet tea, and alcohol.

So what to drink? Water, unsweetened tea, or Crystal Light - anything without calories built in is ideal. We want to spend our food calories on food that gives us something of value.

Visualize food that gives up fullness and nutrition. Liquid calories rarely have the fiber built into whole foods. Tell yourself you will not drink anything with calories.

And, yes, there are exceptions.

Do not drink with your meals

Liquid calories go in and out of the stomach pouch or sleeve very quickly and at best provide a brief sensation of fullness. Have you ever watched an eating contest on TV? The method they use to eat a *gazillion* hot dogs is to drink lots of water in the process. They simply wash the food out of their stomach and into the rest of their gastrointestinal tract, which has lots of room. This is not healthy nor is it the way we were built to eat. It is, however, the way to win the contest.

We need all the calories that we eat to be calories that make us feel full and satisfied for about four hours. We need to eat solid food that makes us full and satisfied with a small volume. Meats that are moist and very chewable are good choices when eaten with a couple small servings of whole foods.

Again, the most important value we can get while eating is getting full and satisfied on a small volume of food that lasts for four hours. I think fullness sends a message to our brain that tells it to burn calories instead of conserving calories. In other words, a different biochemical pathway goes into action.

Avoid carbonated beverages, diet or otherwise

Have you ever noticed all the overweight people who drink diet carbonated soft drinks? Have you also noticed fit people rarely drink diet soft drinks? I do not have a scientific reason to suggest why you should not drink them, but simple observation tells us the diet drinks do not work in our favor.

I think the carbonation tickles the stomach making it less sensitive to fullness and the sweetness drives us to snacking. And more importantly, right or wrong about this theory, this is one of a small number of rules to follow that are associated with success. You need to develop the habit of following the simple rules and not pick and choose. Possibly the most important thing we can do is to learn to give up the resistance to following rules. This is a good time to test your self.

Learn to feel what fullness is

In Chapter 6 I talk about the amygdala and how when we focus on something, we can become very aware of it. So is true with the sensation of fullness. If, for example, we wanted to become more sensitive to touch, we could do so by focusing on touch. Take your index finger-tip and touch things around you. Try to touch softly, then with more force. Think of how something feels and translate that into colors such as red, orange, blue, or green. Very quickly your finger tip touch would become more sensitive. Learning to become aware of the sensation of fullness is just as possible, and it is a very important tool for success.

I remember eating at a fast-food place about twenty years ago with one of my fellow chief residents, who was also a good friend. I sat in amazement as he told me he had never felt full in his life. At the time, I thought that was very odd. It turns out to be common, but in different degrees.

Think in terms of having an ongoing conversation with your stomach, as if it were a friend. Keep asking, "Hey, stomach down there, wake up! How do you feel? Start talking to me. Was that one bite too many?" Pay attention to how being satisfied - but not overly full - feels. Visualize it and tell your brain you want to remember that sensation.

Get comfortable with the wasting food rule

We live in a time of food abundance, yet we have difficulty wasting food. We have to learn to *get comfortable wasting food* to be successful. So at every meal, try wasting some food. Over time the habit becomes easy, but at first there is resistance. No matter how good something tastes, never eat all of it. That inner drive to clean your plate is present in all of us. We blame it on our parents telling us to clean our plate when we were young. However I feel we are hard-wired to do this because of our ancient ancestors, who had to eat all they could eat when it was available because it may not have been available later.

The habit of wasting food will help you learn proper portions to eat. The habit of learning to feel full and satisfied on four to six ounces of food is important for long-term success. It is portion control and it works.

Eat slowly

If you are a fast eater, learning to eat more slowly will take time and practice, and will not happen overnight. It will, however, help you have long-term success and is worth the effort. So what to do? Try letting go of whatever tool you are eating with after every bite, whether it is a spoon or fork, chopsticks, or something you are eating with your hands. Set it down. You will feel an inner sigh of relief and relaxation.

Think of this almost like you are taking recess at school as a child, recess from intensely pursuing your goal. Feel that. Remember that. We tend to be chewing one bite and have the next bite locked and loaded, ready to enter our mouths as soon as we swallow. If setting your utensil or food down for a recess does not get the job done, then try eating with child-size utensils, or better yet, try switching to your non-dominant hand. Switching to your non-dominante hand has the extra benefit of rapidly teaching you to be ambidextrous, while serving the purpose of slowing you down (never mind the fact that it might add a little humor to your meal).

Celebrate your success

These habits do not develop overnight, but stay focused. Chip away at them and celebrate your success of *fitting into those skinny jeans*. You can do it!

5
PITFALLS TO SUCCESS

Gary Chapman's book *The Five Languages of Love,* points out that we basically express our emotional love through five languages: words of affirmation, quality time, receiving gifts, acts of service, and physical touch. This is a very powerful and important relationship concept. It is important to know your personal love language and the language of those you love. We are all the same in that we want to show and receive love. We are different by which language is our own language.

A universal way to show emotional love is through food. Unfortunately, this is a pitfall to long-term weight loss success.

Showing love through food

I have been divorced for eight years now and have a very good relationship with my ex. My kids are getting older now, and good eating habits are fairly well established. Since my divorce, I have had the opportunity to have my kids all to myself. It was all me, and I would find myself trying to show love through food, despite teaching otherwise to my patients.

You see for me, and almost all divorced people, there is guilt. So when we are with our kids, we want to drown them in love. So I would use this desire to buy ice cream, pizza, and all kinds of unhealthy food in preparation for my time with them. Common sense aside, I still felt that strong drive to show love through food - bad food. I would laugh at myself and think, *Are you kidding? What are you doing?* It made me realize how strong the drive is to show love through food. It was not how I would eat otherwise, so the difference was obvious.

Showing love through food is a negative way to show love. Why? It leads to gaining excess weight, which we know is harmful. There are many dysfunctional relationships and we are all probably guilty of showing love in some way that is sometimes harmful. It is important for us to recognize when it happens.

Even without guilt, we live in an age where we try to shower our kids and loved ones with love at every turn. So everybody needs to learn to show love through food in a way that is not harmful.

Mary Ann is your typical busy mother. She is busy working, as well as trying to be a good mother and spouse. She does the grocery shopping. She buys soft drinks, chips, and ice cream. She says they are not for her but the kids. If she does not buy them, then the kids say things like, "There is never any food here."

One of the best tools to prevent snacking is to have shelves and refrigerators empty of bad, unhealthy food. But in doing so, you will face the firing squad. So Mary Ann tells me that she feels like a bad mom when this happens. It is tough love. And in the beginning it hurts. But it is the right thing to do - for them and yourself. At least on a mild level, most people have trouble maintaining a normal weight because we live in a calorie-rich environment.

Emotional eating

Betty is a good mom. Her daughter is struggling with life. She is in trouble with the law and quite possibly going to jail. Betty is nine years out from a gastric bypass and has been very successful at maintaining a healthy weight for those nine years. However, she has recently started regaining weight. She remembered me telling her that if she ever started regaining weight, one of the best things she can do is start making monthly office visits. On her first monthly visit she went through the details of her daughter's tragedy, and began crying. She was starting to snack. She called it emotional eating, and it was her way to show love to herself.

Our brains do not like to be told it cannot have something. In Chapter 6 on inner secrets, I discuss the importance of reframing the language we use to communicate with ourselves and others. We need to reframe our words so that our brain is not being told it cannot have something. So, tell yourself you can have it, but with rules.

Often the person with the snacking problem is the person who does the grocery shopping. The best way to stop snacking is to stop buying snack food. So while shopping, and feeling the urge to buy snack food, pause for a moment and remember what it is like to *fit into those skinny jeans*. Once it is at home, relying on will power to *not* snack will *not work*. If snack food makes it home, consider it eaten unless you can follow the *get comfortable wasting food* rule.

If you make a bad decision at the grocery store and snack food makes it home then you need to eat one helping and enjoy it without blame. Truly enjoy it. Then throw the rest in the trash can. Do it every time. Over time your subconscious will not want to waste anymore food and that decision to *not* buy snack food at the grocery store will no longer be difficut to make. It is magic and it works.

So how do you show love to yourself? Think of the five languages of love. Whether your language is touch, words of affirmation, acts of service, giving a gift, or quality time, give it to yourself in some way that is healthy and not harmful.

Grazing and craving

Grazing on food is a common pitfall for success. Often it is a bite here and a bite there, all day long. This is a recipe for failure with any weight loss surgery we do. Journaling is a good method to make you aware that grazing is happening, and awareness is the first step to all change. Once aware, go to work trying to find a solution to the problem, which in general is either not buying it or eating one helping and wasting the rest.

You will not be graded on your journaling. It is for you alone. The hardest person to be honest with is you. Once you have achieved awareness, then maybe you can forgo journaling. Until then, make a rule to write down everything that goes into your mouth. Be truthful. Every bite counts. Your journal is a tool.

For many the work place has a common area always full of food laid out and ready for the *passing-by nibbler*. This makes it difficult not to snack. Instead of telling the snack bringers they are doing something bad, talk about how it feels to *fit into those skinny jeans* and why success requires no snacking.

It is impossible to change others who do not want to change. Mentoring works by showing others what success looks like. As they see your healthiness, vitality, and all those things that make up the essence of *fitting into those skinny jeans*, they just might be willing to change.

Beyong grazing, we sometimes get a strong craving for certain food, say chocolate. But it could be bread, chips, ice cream, or almost anything. Never keep the food that you sometimes crave at home. If you must have it, then get dressed, get in your car and go someplace and get one helping and eat it there. Enjoy it, embrace the moment, but do not bring it home. Over time that craving will disappear.

In general, we are subconsciously too lazy to do it often enough for it to matter in terms of long-term weight loss success. Think of this process as a tool.

Drinking with your meals

We digest food better if we do not drink while eating, but it has become customary to drink while eating. Doing this washes the food rapidly out of our stomach before adequate digestion and before adequate fullness occurs. It is a difficult custom to break. So here is a tool. Do not keep anything to drink next to your plate. If you have a strong desire to drink while eating, get up from the table and go to the kitchen. Take one drink, then go and sit back down to your meal. Keep doing this every time you feel the need to have a drink. Over time that need will disappear like magic.

At a restaurant it is difficult not having a glass of something next to your plate. The waiters will keep asking if they can get you something and it gets annoying. Hopefully, though, you will spend most of your eating time not in restaurants and can establish this habit.

Skipping meals

Believe it or not skipping meals is a pitfall. To our brains, it seems to make sense that if we eat, we get fat; and if we do not eat, we lose weight. Years and years of starvation diets have shown the same result. We lose weight at first, but as soon as we stop starving, we regain weight rapidly and with a vengeance, usually everything we lost plus a ten percent gain. We have all tried it and we all know it to be true.

It seems intuitively backwards that we need to eat to maintain a healthy weight, but it is true. I think we need a small volume of food and the sensation of satisfied fullness to send messages to the brain to burn not conserve calories.

I personally prefer not to eat breakfast. I am usually ready to start my day and do not want to waste time. But I remind myself almost every day that it is important to eat a small breakfast. Many weight loss surgery patients get very full, very easily in the morning, and it is very easy for them to skip breakfast. However, they need to at least eat something to get their metabolism headed in the right direction - burning calories versus storing calories. It is something we learned in medicine many years ago. That's when the sugar dextrose was added to basic intravenous solutions. Think of it as a scale much like the scale of justice. On one side of the scale our metabolism burns calories: on the other side of the scale, it conserves calories. The biochemical pathways that burn calories require calories to prime the process. So, eat breakfast and do not skip meals.

These are the most common pitfalls that I hear from patients who are struggling with success. I have tried to keep them few and straight forward. There are other pitfalls. Try to learn the process of identifying your personal pitfalls and then coming up with a tool or method to give your brain what it wants without it being harmful to long-term success.

Skinny Jeans....At Last

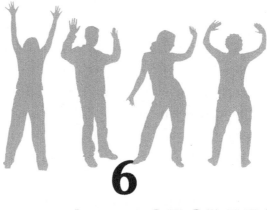

6
INNER SELF SECRETS

*Start by trying to feel your gift and how you want
to give your gift to the world*

-Clifton Thomas, MD

We have all seen those undercover TV programs where a journalist dresses up in a fat suit and goes about their day. For a moment in their lives they get a chance to walk in your shoes. They get to feel, really feel those moments where they are treated differently because they are fat. And it hurts. It hurts deeply and affects our inner self.

I have never walked in your shoes. I am not a behavioral modification specialist. What I have done is listen. And feel. As I listen, I try to think of things I have learned that help me and will hopefully help you. We could all benefit from working on our inner selves - fat or not.

I rarely use the word "fat". Why? Well, it is harsh and carries with it that sense of discrimination. It feels wrong. The words we choose when talking to ourselves and others matter. That's where I would like to begin this chapter: talking about how we can dramatically change by adjusting the words we use. This chapter is about change.

We are who we are. I believe that. I believe we all have an inner gift that is very special. It is who we are, that *thing* that is you. It is your soul. It is the core of your personality. We often bury it very deep, and what people feel is not your gift, but years and years of unhappiness and bitterness from years and years of discrimination. This chapter is about uncovering your gift.

I have to share something that has amused me and pleases me very much. As I look at patients roughly a year out from surgery who have lost about one hundred pounds I cannot visualize what they looked like before surgery. But I feel like I know them. Of course I can remember when I look back at pictures, but not when sitting in front of them. I think I see their gift instead, that very special thing that is them.

The goal of this chapter is to share some concepts that will help you tap into your gift so that you may be able to give your gift to the world and live a life of fulfillment.

Weight loss surgery dramatically changes the dynamics in your life. We should all focus on controlling what we *can* control. And we can control the way we change - the direction we change.

> **Start by trying to feel your gift and how you want to give that to the world.**

Visualize where you have been and where you want your life to go. Get a real sense of what that is and never let go of it. Understand that by physically feeling better, being more productive, by having more self-confidence, you will be more able to give your gift . Never let that go. Hold onto it forever.

Every day visualize and celebrate what you have accomplished. Do this and you will stay focused and have that secret to long-term weight loss surgery success.

This chapter is not complete. It is simply me sharing some concepts that I am familiar with. Know where you want your life to go and go on a path that allows you to give your gift to the world. Stay aligned with that path. Any time you get off track, look for a tool or concept to help you get back on your path.

We live in an age of information good and bad. Find the good information that is congruent with your path and will allow you to give your gift. If your car is badly out of alignment you will have difficulty getting where you want to go. Stay in alignment.

We have an amazing brain. It has an area called the amygdala, which is responsible for filtering all of our senses. It lets some in and keeps others out. When we focus on a problem and start seriously looking to solve it, our amygdala filters that information, and ta-da, we magically find and fix it.

For example, if we visualize finding a parking space close to a particular business, our amygdala will get busy filtering all kinds of subconscious information. We sense the flow of traffic, which aisle to check, which not to check, and ta-da! We find that special parking space. This is all working subconsciously because you focused on it and the amygdala got busy. This example is an over simplification but you get the point: There are tools available to you when your path is out of alignment.

> **Get aligned. Find the problem. Fix it.**
> **And give your gift to the world.**

The words we use when talking to ourselves and others are very important. I am not talking about political correctness here, but something very different.

Visualize for a moment being burned by fire as a child. Visualize the pain and the scars. Try to feel for a moment what that feels like. Now try to visualize never being burned by fire. Instead, everything you remember about fire involves those warm fuzzy moments where you, family, friends or lovers are sitting around a fire, feeling the warmth of the flames and of those with you.

The word *fire* when spoken, read, or thought will immediately send chemicals like adrenaline or oxytocin through your body, changing your physiology (the way you feel). The fastest most effective way to change the way you feel immediately is to adjust the words we use to ourselves and others.

Neurolinguistic Programming, NLP, is an amazing and complex area of study. Many years ago I read *Mindlines: Lines for Changing Minds,* a book by the founders of NLP, Michael Hall and Bodenhamer. It is a difficult read, though I found the concept simple and profound. There is both a dark side to NLP and a bright side. Practitioners of NLP can easily manipulate people. That is not what I want you to learn. What I want you to understand and learn is that the words you use to talk yourself and others are critically important for change.

Recently I was driving to a restaurant in Houston with my girlfriend, who is familiar with NLP. I was taking the route I knew. She thought she knew a better way and probably *did* know a better way. But I was the driver and we were together to be together.

I could sense her frustration, but being a typical guy, I did not like being told "turn here, turn there."

NLP practioners use the term *reframing*. In this situation I asked my girlfriend to re-frame her thoughts of how I was taking the wrong path to the restaurant to thoughts of something different.

So, she began thinking differently and - different words started coming from the voices inside her head: *the longer we take, the longer we are sitting close, side by side, holding hands, feeling each other's warmth and love*. All true. All congruent with our relationship.

Pay attention to how you feel on the inside as you talk to yourself and to others. I this is not congruent with your gift then change the words you use and change your life.

Suffering is a part of what we experience. Birth, aging, illness, despair, pain, and grief are examples of times we suffer. It is a part of life. It is built into almost everything. We should focus on what we can control. We can control how much we suffer.

The Four Noble Truths, as passed down by Buddha, give us insight to happiness, fulfillment, pain, and suffering. Shin Zen Young took this concept further by adding that suffering is the result of resisting pain. Think of it as a formula; Pain x Resistance = Suffering.

We are all going to experience pain, but the amount we suffer is optional. If we resist the pain - the suffering will increase. The secret is to learn to give up the resistance and embrace the pain, not an easy task and not one that will happen overnight. We need to begin by understanding the concept. Once we understand and can feel how resistance adds to our suffering we can go to work on changing suffering.

Suffering is a very strong emotion. We feel emotion. The feeling comes from chemicals that are released inside our bodies. We can become addicted to those chemicals.

Giving up our resistance to following simple eating rules and changing the environment that triggers our addiction allows us to have long-term weight loss surgery success.

How do we give up resistance? Go back to Chapter 3. Read the stories. Feel the emotion of what it is like to *fit into those skinny jeans...at last!* Then tell yourself, *if I was given a million dollars to plan when and what I was going to eat and follow that plan it would be the easiest million ever.* Then do it. Do it year after year, and it will become who you are.

Also ask yourself, *if I was given a million dollars to change the environment that triggers my addiction, could I do that?* I think you can. This is much more challenging than giving up the resistance to following simple eating rules.

But how do you change your environment? Say, for example, you enjoy drinking wine each evening with your spouse. It is one of those moments you just seem to connect. But you drink more than a glass night after night. Well, long-term weight loss surgery success is not possible, unless you change that environment.

Start by not buying or bringing home wine. If it makes it home somehow, then drink one glass, enjoy it, and then waste the rest of the bottle. Throw it away. Over time your subconscious will not like wasting wine, and the wine will somehow no longer make it home. Drink, enjoy, and waste, every time. Recall the *get comfortable with wasting food* rule in Chapter 5.

It may be that you enjoy eating ice cream while sitting on the couch watching your favorite TV program with your spouse - well the same applies. Find another way to connect. Try walking and talking while enjoying the beauty of the outdoors. These are simple examples; more complex examples exist in dysfunctional relationships with friends, families, or co-workers. They enable bad eating habits. And, no, you cannot waste *them.*

Divorce is very high following weight loss surgery. Divorce is very high after any major life changing event. Remember we show love through food, but it is the wrong way to show love because it leads to suffering from being overweight. It is difficult to talk about bad eating habits with your spouse. The best way to get them to change is by mentoring. Show them how you eat, day after day.

My daughter spent a year as a Rotary exchange student in Brazil. After about nine months, I went to visit. When I got off the plane I was shocked to see that she had gained significant weight. Prior to the exchange, she had never been anythiing but slim and trim. Of course I was smart enough to keep my thoughts to myself.

I quickly realized what was going on - it was her environment. The first restaurant we ate at served us a huge plate with multiple pieces of steak. It was only my daughter, her friend and I, but somehow we finished it. Before long they brought another plate of food. I forced myself to eat more and, sure enough, felt tired and bloated from overeating. My daughter was eating more than she normally would because she felt it was rude not to eat the food they brought her.

It was their way of showing love. So I ate that way as well for several days before deciding I was done overeating. From that point on, I would politely only eat one reasonable helping of food.

At the end of the two-week trip, my daughter's exchange father came up to me and said that he had been watching the way I ate and was going to start eating that way as well. He had developed high blood pressure and was feeling bad.

Mentoring, showing others by example, works.

If mentoring does not work then maybe changing your exposure to the dysfunctional friends, families, or co-workers is in order. Addiction to suffering is not easy to resolve. You must focus on it, give up the resistance to change, and change your environment.

By the way, after one year my daughter came home and returned to her normal eating habits and quickly returned to her normal weight. How? She changed her environment.

> **Willpower is not a character issue.**
> **Our brains are simply not designed for**
> **willpower.**

Most of us assume that if we do not have the will power to do something it is a character weakness that can be overcome. But research clearly shows that our brains simply aren't designed for willpower: in fact willpower is a limited resource in the brain.

A series of experiments has clearly demonstrated that the part of the brain responsible for self-control - the prefrontal cortex - simply can't maintain the act of self-control for an extended period of time.

These experiments were performed by Baba Shiv, a Stanford University professor. One part of the experiment assembled two groups. One group was asked to remember a two-digit number, the other group was asked to remember a seven-digit number. Then both groups were given the choice of eating a bowl of healthy fruit salad or a very unhealthy slice of cake.

The seven digit number group was twice as likely to eat the cake. The reason is the prefrontal cortex (the part of the brain responsible for self-control) was overloaded with remembering the seven digits.

Will power is a limited resource in the brain and cannot be maintained for an extended period of time, therefore tools are needed to change eating habits.

> **It is common to sacrifice long term gains**
> **for short term satisfaction.**

I was at the movie theater recently and planned to buy a snack before the movie. Near the counter was a small bag of frozen, M-&-M-size ice cream bites. I thought, *This looks good, I deserve it.* I flipped the package over and read with amazement. It contained 25 grams of saturated fat per serving.

At the very best, eating that treat would have given me a very brief moment of satisfaction.

So, I put it back. I know that I cannot eat that way without long term consequences. Every day we need to ask ourselves whether we are sacrificing long-term weight loss surgery success for short-term satisfaction. We know the answer - what we can't do is ignore the question. We need to ask the question every time, every day. Like magic the need for the question will disappear.

7

THE NUMBER ONE SECRET TO STAYING IN THOSE SKINNY JEANS

The secret to staying in those skinny jeans is *staying focused* for the rest of your life.

The two variables most responsible for our obesity - our genetics and our calorie-rich environment - are not likely to change. So it is vital that the feeling of What it is like to *fit into those skinny jeans* become an ever present thought.

What does staying focused look like? Allison had a gastric bypass nine years ago and has kept her eighty-five pounds off. She has a small frame, so eighty-five pounds is a lot. She is gorgeous, and often gets compliments on her appearance.

Allison has faithfully kept all of her doctor follow-up appointments. If you find someone that had a gastric bypass or sleeve gastrectomy that has regained significant weight, ask them, "When was the last time you saw your bariatric surgeon?" Almost always you will get a vague answer full of excuses.

We teach all patients that one of the best things they can do if they begin to regain significant weight is to start seeing their bariatric surgeon monthly until they are back on track. The act of scheduling the appointment, arranging time to make the appointment, walking in, waiting, and sitting in the exam room keeps those inner voices actively thinking about weight loss.

From there, we can focus our discussion about what part of the eating rules they are struggling with and what to do about it. Patients are often afraid that I am going to be disappointed in them. I am not. I know how challenging it is. I am disappointed, however, when I hear of a patient regaining weight and not coming to the office.

Allison volunteers in all kinds of civic organizations. She frequently has to eat at various luncheons and the like. She goes to bed at night and plans her next eating day. She visualizes when and what she will eat and has healthy backup food available just in case. This keeps her focused.

Within the first year following her surgery, Allison found a personal trainer and started exercising regularly. The act of scheduling the workout, - the fact that someone was expecting her at a specific time, and the fact that it cost hard-earned-money - kept her accountable. Over time she made a friend at the gym, and they started working out together. They made a pact to keep each other accountable. Punches allowed.

Allison is a walking advertisement for weight loss surgery. She talks about weight loss surgery and it keeps her focused. She realizes people are watching her - the way she eats and the choices she makes. She is a good mentor for anyone watching. Her kids have said thing like, "There is never any food in the house," which could make her feel like she is a bad mom. She, too, has an inner drive to show love to her kids by giving them unhealthy snacks; however, she learned to show her love differently - the tough way.

Allison actively participates in our online support group. Just the act of sitting down at the computer at a specified time, logging in, and listening, helps her stay focused. Sometimes she hears or shares something of importance, and sometimes not. Just the act of doing this helps keep her focused.

It is very easy to lose the excess weight and feel the problem is gone - to feel excited about becoming attractive and have the energy for fun. It is also very easy to then begin acting just like those around you, eating carelessly, going to happy hour, eating the ever present food that surrounds us because that is what everyone else is doing. If we do that, guess what? The skinny jeans no longer fit!

Most weight loss books use the majority of their pages to explain some theory concerning the type of food we should eat.

We have not - for a reason.

The reason is that the most important task to learn is to follow *some* eating rules. Once that is accomplished, it is time to fine-tune your eating habits, learn about the nutritional content of food, and become an expert on healthy eating.

And interestingly - in my opinion - the most important thing that this accomplishes is staying focused. You will be conscious of what you put into your mouth, and it will carry you further up the ladder to healthiness.

Staying focused, following simple, doable eating rules, and giving up the resistance to doing them is *the secret* to long-term weight loss surgery success.

Skinny Jeans....At Last

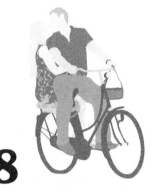

8

CALORIES, ZOO ANIMALS AND THOSE BATHROOM SCALES

The most valuable thing you can do for your long-term health is to eat healthy. The longer you do it, the more you realize it's true.

-Clifton Thomas, MD

We as humans feel we can dump anything into our gastrointestinal tract and it can handle it. Look around and observe animal eating behavior and think back to early man. Does this make sense, or should we be eating a specialized diet? And do we really have the knowledge to know what specialized diet we should be eating? While that could be a book in itself, this book is about the mindset for long-term weight loss success.

This chapter is a mix of subjects with the underlining purpose of shifting your primary mindset to one of observation and awareness of how your body responds to eating behaviors.

For long-term success you need to tune into your body and observe how it responds. I recommend trying something different and seeing how you feel - the trial-and-error approach.

Zoo animals are in captivity, living in some incomplete semblance of their environment. The most important thing for their survival is their diet - what they eat. Zoo-keepers have learned from their mistakes and so have we. Methods of detecting nutritional deficiencies are getting better, but most of our knowledge of nutrition comes from trial and error.

For example, the early explorers who sailed the world learned by trial and error that they would need to carry fruit on the ships or the sailors would develop scurvy.

> **We as humans need to look at what we eat,**
> **tune in to how our body responds,**
> **and realize we cannot just dump *anything***
> **into our gastrointestinal tract**
> **and wake up feeling good.**

It is nearly impossible to recreate the zoo animal's natural diet, and as a result, captive animals develop more illnesses like heart disease, renal problems, and diabetes - than those in the wild. Zoo-keepers obtain food for the animals much like we do, from grocery store distributors. Their variety of fruit, for example, is similar to ours.

Because these store-bought fruits have much more sugar and less fiber than fruits in the wild, some frui- eating animals like the binturongs develop diabetes. The food fed to zoo animals is "people quality" and, as a consequence, it needs to be fortified.

Certain animals in the wild eat only bark from trees and shrubs. Yet they still grow large and active, and are healthy because they are consuming the nutritional calories they require. They eat food they have evolved to eat.

When we feed our dogs from the table - once again showing love through food - we are doing them more harm than good. Over time they develop human-like illnesses. Have you ever seen a dog that is only fed high-quality dog food and observed how lean and healthy they look? Compare that with dogs that are fed kitchen scraps.

Advice on what we should eat or the supplements we should take is abundant. But what do we really know about nutrition, and how did we learn it?

We learned most of what we know much like the zoo keepers did. In the early 1970s, we began feeding tiny, immature babies through intravenous nutrition and pretty rapidly had some success. Then we started using intravenous nutrition called TPN to feed adults who could not be fed by mouth. We started off giving what we thought was necessary, mostly sugar - estimating what we thought a person needed for whatever medical condition they had. We soon found that too much sugar caused lots of problems.

We started adding protein and then we learned that too much and not enough was a problem.

We started noticing severe skin conditions that turned out to be a fat deficiency and we started adding fats. Many other medical issues occurred and we learned to add vitamins and minerals. We also found out what happened when we gave too much and what happened when we gave too little.

That's where the learning began. Most of what we now know came from those mistakes. And it is true that most of what we all know in every endeavor comes from learning from our mistakes. We learned what medical issues occurred when certain things were not given.

We learned from our mistakes.

Believe it or not the same is true today. The science that tells us what to eat, in relative terms, is weak - that's why there are so many different opinions and diets, the pyramid system, the low carbohydrate diets like Atkins and South Beach, the Mediterranean diets ... The list goes on. We still have the same problem and really the same solution to the problem, that we had in the early 1970s: What should we eat?

Even to this day, we have poor methods of measuring our metabolism and knowing how many calories we need to burn. We guess when it comes to supplements. We are just starting to get laboratory methods for measuring nutrient needs. To do this properly we need to measure very specifically what goes into our mouths, find better ways to test what is happening in the body and measure what happens later in terms of our physical well-being. We need to know better what is absorbed, what is not, and why.

We are getting closer to doing just this, but we still have a very long way to go.

The abundance of information is guessing from the knowledge of chemical pathways in our bodies and assuming that if some chemical is needed for a pathway - if we take it as a supplement - our GI tract will absorb it and use it. There are a lot of assumptions.

I want to applaud all the amazing work done by brilliant scientists and physicians in the area of nutrition. In some areas the science explaining how we get a certain nutrient is good and in some areas it is weak.

> **For long-term weight loss surgery success, it's very important to take the recommended supplements summarized in the addendum.**

These examples are generalizations that make a point. The point I am trying to make is that we need to take the best advice, try it, but then see how our body responds, and do laboratory tests for correlation. I like one called NutrEval by Genova Diagnostics. We need to pay attention to what we eat and pay attention to how our bodies respond, whether it is fast food, grocery store food, or health-food supplements.

We focus on calories. I am sure it is surprising for most to know how poor the science is behind what a food calorie is and, more importantly, how little we know about how that relates to our metabolism and body functions.

We do know that a calorie is the amount of energy in terms of heat released when a particular food is burned in a bomb calorimeter. We know our bodies do not burn calories like a bomb calorimeter. Yet everything about food calories is based on the basic knowledge obtained from a bomb calorimeter.

Even then mathematical models take that information and extrapolate it to all foods. In other words, very few of the foods we eat and the calories on the label have actually been tested in a bomb calorimeter.

I do not mean to insult the brilliant scientists who have spent their careers developing this useful information. But it reminds me of the global warming issue: The science that blames us humans for significantly impacting global warming is poor.

That said, I think it does bring into the spotlight the need to be responsible humans and take care of our planet. We also seem to learn the most about how to take care of our planet from our mistakes. Counting calories is important in general, but not in specific terms. It is important to know roughly how many calories are in certain foods and roughly how many calories we need to function well.

Recently I was thinking of buying a box of peanut butter Girl Scout Cookies. I flipped the box over and read the label. There were 150 calories per cookie. I handed the box back and gave a donation. Why? I know myself.

I could not eat just one and get much enjoyment out of it. Instead, I would need to sit down with a glass of milk, dip each cookie in the milk and quickly eat it. And in very little time I would have eaten the majority of the box, which would have been several thousand calories. Clearly not smart.

> **I think of calories like money.**

Money is just a piece of paper with symbols on it that varies in purchasing power. We should be thinking in terms of what money can buy today, and how much value it gives us. We know the problem is not the expensive things we buy (they give us great value). It's the pennies we spend on short-term satisfaction and very little long-term value. It's the *expensive, super-duper everything-in-it* drive-through coffee.

Calories, like money, are important. And we should have a general idea of how many calories we need and spend those with value. And we should be thinking in terms of long-term benefits versus short-term satisfaction.

So how do we know what we should eat and how much? We should use the method proven by the test of time. That is, learn from our mistakes. I am going to tell you how to do that, but first I would like to back up to our talk on zoo animals and talk about our ancestors, who were hunters and gatherers.

Zookeepers determine the animals' diets by looking at their environment and behavior in the wild, not in the zoo. Then they recreate it the best they can, see what works, and change what does not work. The genetics that control the bio-chemical pathways in our bodies have evolved over time, but there is no evidence they have significantly changed since the dawn of agriculture.

I think it is important to look back at ancient times and ask, *What did early man eat to survive?* There may be some argument as to exactly what that was, but it is safe to assume that ancient humans hunted for meat and gathered food. It most likely consisted of lean meats, leafy greens, fruit, berries, and seeds. The majority of their energy went into hunting and gathering food. Their survival depended on it. Food was scarce and difficult to obtain.

I believe their genetic bio-chemical pathways told their bodies that something was very wrong when food was not available and would shut down the *burning calorie* metabolism. They would eat when food was available, most likely until they were full. It is my belief that fullness, not over fullness, tells our brains to burn calories.

> **Starvation, including low calorie diets, tell our brains to shut down our metabolism and store calories.**

Many years ago I read a book called *The Food Chronology* by James Trager. It discusses our earliest knowledge of early humans and examines what evidence there is about what they ate. The book then marches through historical events up to present time. It matches historical events with what was going on in relation to food at the time.

Skimming through the book, you can get a tremendous sense of how we have arrived where we are today. And it brings us back to learning from our mistakes.

When farming became a trade, wheat and grains were the main crop. Then came the major plagues, which killed millions of people because rodents ate the stock-piled grains, multiplied rapidly and spread disease. The naturopathic doctors have brought into the spotlight how common gluten sensitivity is and how it adversely affects our health.

Gastroenterologists missed the boat when it comes to gluten sensitivity. They focused on celiac disease, which is the severe form of gluten sensitivity, and ignored the minor effects gluten sensitivity caused in terms of intestinal symptoms, such as cramps, constipation, diarrhea, bloating, skin rashes, migraines, nasal congestion and autoimmune disease, to name a few.

I now recommend to any patient having any type of GI problems that they do a brief trial of a gluten-free diet. And I am amazed how many people report back that their health has significantly improved. If you don't believe me, try it. Ask your friends who have some of the above problems to do the gluten-free diet and have them report back how they feel. You will be amazed.

Back to the topic of wheat, it is widely touted that grains are very healthy, that we should eat oatmeal, wheat bread and cereals. But they cause many people to have problems. So if you go through a gluten-free trial and find that in many ways you feel better, then step back and observe the abundance of information there has been that wheat is healthy. You might be getting the idea that much of the advice we get regarding diet is not as solid as we think.

For example, we learned that we need a lot of fiber in our diet. We thought that because wheat has a lot of fiber it must be healthy and that we should be eating it every day. For many it is not. Individuals need to see how they respond to wheat. And if they don't respond well, they should avoid it. Tune in to your body and observe how it responds. Remember there is a lot of fiber in whole foods.

Don't juice them, eat them.

You can follow the posture of homo sapiens through time and see how it has changed since we started bringing laboratory chemistry into our daily lives with plastics, food additives, and refined foods like flour, salt, and sugar.

Our posture has changed for the worse, a change that coincides with the development of food additives and the proliferation of refined foods. While this is not the scientific way to make a conclusion, it appears true to me that we have too many chemicals in our diets.

Food additives are chemicals and have side-effect profiles just like medicines. Just like medicine they affect some and not others. The problem is that there are so many of them laced in our packaged food products that it is difficult to separate those that you can and cannot tolerate. Intuitively it makes sense that some may be causing problems.

Go additive free and see how your body responds

I am going to give you the best proper diet book ever written, now, within this book, as a free bonus, with all the best scientific and best guess information, synthesized down to a brief passage.

Eat a variety of non-packaged whole foods and lean meats preferably from free range animals. No packaged food. No refined flours or foods made from refined flours, like bread and pasta. No refined sugars or salt. You get salt and sugar naturally in whole foods.

Then test yourself. Eat this way completely from Monday through Friday. Then on the weekend go back to eating as usual. Go out to eat and over-eat. Eat the pasta. Eat salty fatty food. Eat packaged food. Write down how you feel Friday morning and again when you wake up Sunday morning. The difference will be dramatic.

If we were given a million dollars to eat this way every day we would find it the easiest million ever. It is simple, maybe too simple. We as humans want a complex solution to a complex problem, like magic supplements.

We like to blame the puffiness and fog-headedness, the poor texture of our skin, the brittleness of our bones, on age. It is mostly our diet. The key is to give up the resistance to eating this way and focus on the benefits and long-term gains. When the resistance is gone....the battle is won.

But what about spaghetti and meat balls? You mean I can't ever eat this again? No, I do not. Once a week or several times a month would be well tolerated without long-term negative effects. But do not make it part of what you eat every day.

I believe that trial and error with our bodies, like our planet, has taught us that they have self-healing abilities and can tolerate brief, limited pollution. If it's more than brief and more than limited, it causes problems.

The most valuable thing you can do for your long-term health is to eat healthy. The longer you do it, the more you will realize it's true.

Expectations

I would now like to talk about expectations. Expectations are important for goal setting and to avoid all those negative inner voices that might defeat us. So what are our expectations when it comes to exercise and getting on the bathroom scale?

Exercise is really bad at helping us lose weight. Picture yourself on a treadmill working very hard and sweating profusely. We can easily imagine that the amount of sweat should equal the amount of pounds falling off. But day after day of stepping on the bathroom scales leads to disappointment and bewilderment. We look at the scale and ask *why?*

> **The scale tells us nothing. It just sits there pointing at the same number.**

Exercise, along with losing weight and maintaining a healthy weight, is very important to our long-term quality of life. It makes us fit to enjoy life more fully. It improves our mental well-being and is excellent at relieving stress. Exercise is all about developing a habit. I think it takes one to two years to develop the habit to the point that you no longer have to talk yourself into exercising.

Visualize yourself paying for an expensive gym membership, driving to the gym and then sitting in the car trying to talk yourself out of going in. Suddenly, everything seems more important than exercising.

The same is true when we try to develop good eating habits. Visualize and remind yourself over and over the things you notice about yourself when you are exercising on a regular basis. Use that visualization to help you give up the resistance to doing the simple, doable things, like getting out of your car and walking into the gym. And give up equating sweating and intensity of exercise with weight loss. If you don't, you will be disappointed and quit. Do not quit. Develop the habit and the intensity can come later.

The two most important tools for success are finding the time of day that is least likely to be interrupted and building some method of accountability.

For some, it's doing a form of exercise first thing in the morning before the hectic day starts. For others, it's finding a partner and agreeing to make each other accountable. If they have an excuse to not show up, give them a hard time, every time.

How about those bathroom scales? I think they give more bad information than good. In a hospital setting we weigh patients daily. It is not because we think they are metabolizing fat and muscle or gaining fat and muscle. It is because we want to know what their water balance is. If the weight increases over night we know they are retaining fluid/water for some reason, and the reverse is true as well.

Scales are useful at home, however, for the same reason. It measures our water balance. I only recommend weighing yourself if you feel as though you are retaining fluid. If your weight goes up overnight, you are. You did not grow fat, or muscle, or bone. It could be for hormonal reasons such as menstrual periods, some medical problem, or side effects of some medicine. But most likely it is because you have been eating salty food.

Most people are salt sensitive and will retain water after eating salty food. They will gain water weight that can be seen on the scale and felt in the puffiness of their fingers.

Prove it to yourself. Eat salt free from Monday to Friday, eat salty food Friday and Saturday, and see how you feel when you wake up Sunday. Then visualize how you felt Monday to Friday and remember that feeling. The next time you think about eating salty food, stop and ask yourself, is it worth it? Learning the nutritional value of food, learning to count calories, learning about metabolic rates and glycemic indexes all are very good.

There are many books on the subject and I highly recommend one from a friend of mine, Robert Moore, called *The Body of Knowledge System.*

This chapter was about the process of tuning into our bodies, and observing how we feel when we eat or don't eat certain foods. Use that emotion as a tool to help you give up the resistance and do it.

The process is safe, cheap, and simple.

You can do it! And it does work.

Skinny Jeans....At Last

9

BYPASS, SLEEVE, OR BAND?

Why do they work?

What's right for me?

Barry Swartz, the author of *The Paradox of Choice,* points out that we live in a world full of choices and that having so many choices causes anxiety.

He points out that one way to reduce that anxiety is to have a clear picture of your goal. (The goal is successful long-term weight loss). He also says to be careful on choosing based on emotion, which I will talk about later.

Almost all patients blame themselves for not being able to lose weight on their own. In most of our human history food was not abundant and we had to work hard to find enough food to survive. The body's chemical pathways are complex and, in my opinion, were evolved during a time when food was not abundant and the danger of starving was very real. We now live in a time of food abundance.

DNA is incredibly amazing. It contains molecules called bases. These four bases, and how they are arranged within the DNA complex, are responsible for the different ways all living things look. People look different because of their DNA. The way DNA is expressed is influenced by its environment. We can look at identical twins who grew up in different families, for example, and if one is obese, so is the other. It is their genetics.

The problem is our genetics and our calorie-rich environment - two variables not easy to change. You need a tool. The only proven tool to work long term is weight loss surgery.

So which is the right procedure for you?

It is the procedure that will give you long-term weight loss success with the least possible risk. One must also consider the risk of failing to achieve long-term weight loss success. In other words, all of those serious medical problems and day-to-day difficulties will not go away if you fail. And that is serious.

I want to talk about how we as surgeons make surgical decisions. I will give you my take on each procedure and why they work, and later how to pick what is right for you.

We think of the patient and their medical problems, the risk of doing a test or an operation, and the benefits of having that information or the benefits of that surgery. A risky test or operation would require lots of benefits to be the right choice.

When having some type of abdominal operation, like a hysterectomy, people often ask if the appendix can be taken out at the same time to prevent future appendicitis? Well, most patients having a hysterectomy are forty years old or older. The risk of developing appendicitis in that age group is one in 70,000.

If a surgeon did 70,000 incidental appendectomies most likely at least one would have a complication related to surgery. The risk, although low, is not worth the benefit of preventing that rare case of appendicitis.

Being able to look at risk and benefits is also useful in everyday life. You are about to take a trip from Houston to Miami. You can drive or fly. Flying is safer than driving. There is less risk of a plane crash than a car accident. Driving is dangerous, but we do it every day. We become numb to the risk, but it is real. What are the benefits of flying versus driving?

Well, first you need a clear picture of your goal. Do you need to get there fast? Is there bad weather that may cancel your flight? Consider all of the many hassles of getting to the airport, parking, checking in, going through security, and waiting for your plane.

Driving creates issues of wear and tear on your car. Also, it would take longer to get there, but would be more of a sure deal. It would be less likely that weather would interfere with you getting there and being able to return home as planned. For some, you also need to factor in a fear of flying.

As Barry Schwartz pointed out - be careful on choosing based on emotion.

Pick the winning option
by having a clear picture of your goal.
Do not make the decision based on emotional fear.

The gastric bypass is a complex operation. The more complex an operation, the more opportunities there are for things to go wrong. This is true for all surgeries and for anything mechanical.

Surgeons with comprehensive bariatric practices have documented low complication rates. Currently, those risks are even lower than those associated with gallbladder surgery. But they are real, and if they occur, it is a big deal for the patient, the family, and the surgeon.

The **gastric bypass** has the lowest failure rate. It does more of the work for you. During a gastric bypass the upper part of the stomach is divided from the rest of stomach. This shot-glass-size part of the stomach is then connected to the upper part of the small intestine. So food goes into this small-size stomach, into the small intestine, into the large intestines, and after digestion and fermentation to the toilet.

Food does not go into the other greater-size portion of the stomach, or into the second portion of the intestine called the duodenum. Food bypasses these areas. As I mentioned earlier, there are many chemicals in this area that work by biofeedback. The way they affect our body metabolism changes because food did not pass through that area or bypassed that area of the intestine.

These chemical changes are the magic.

The magic of the way the gastric bypass is the most effective tool - that is - why it does more of the work for you.

The gastric bypass probably still has an edge on the sleeve gastrectomy in diabetic patients, but time will tell. Most diabetic patients who have a gastric bypass are off insulin within the first week after surgery and often the first night of surgery. This is absolutely amazing and due to those chemical changes that normalize our metabolism.

The **sleeve gastrectomy** had its beginnings around 2003, but it has only recently become popular and approved by many insurance companies. The more we do it the better the results get. Recent five-year studies now show it to be equally as effective as the gastric bypass. It seems to have many, if not all of the chemical changes we get with the gastric bypass - the chemical changes that normalize our metabolism and make it easier to choose healthy eating habits. The operation is less complex than the gastric bypass, and less complexity translates into fewer complications.

During a sleeve gastrectomy, the upper portion of the stomach is turned into a tube shape by removing about two-thirds of the stomach. The lower third, the antrum, is left untouched. Patients feel full on a small volume of food. But the magic is in the chemical changes.

I started doing the **lap band** November 2002. It was approved by the FDA in June 2002. At first I had doubts about the band's long-term success. I was afraid it would have the same outcome as the vertical banded gastroplasty of the 1980s with it's high failure rate.

I attended a master's course at our society meeting. After a pro-and-con session, the question was asked, "OK, surgeons, if it were you which oper-ation would you chose?" Repeatedly, seasoned gastric bypass surgeons ap-proached the microphone and said, "I would choose the band because of less risk of complications".

It made sense that patients should have the choice to pick the amount of risk they are willing to tolerate to accomplish their goals. It is, however, just as important to factor in the risk of failure and its harmful effects.

I have lots of band success stories. And I probably have more band failures than I realize.

The band is nothing more than an inner tube placed around the upper part of the stomach. We add saline to the inner tube to make it tighter. We take saline out if it is too tight. The stomach above the band is not like a black box. It is pliable like a balloon. It is dynamic. It changes like a balloon.

However, most patients get full and satisfied on four to six ounces of food. The amount of food it takes to get full varies with the time of day, your emotional status, and other reasons we don't understand.

**Patients who find success with the band
are people who are very good at planning
and following rules and in their daily lives.**

Often they are a little obsessive about following their daily plan and get a little anxious if it is not happening. They find success easy and wonder why more people do not do better.

Well, most people live their lives with good intentions, but most of their days are lived haphazardly. Patients must learn to follow the eating rules first. Success will follow.

With the gastric bypass and the sleeve, the operation forces patients to follow rules in the beginning. Later on they must develop their own eating rule habits to have long-term success.

The chemical changes that normalize metabolism do not occur with band surgery. The band is the least complicated operation and has the fewest complications. But it has the highest failure rate.

To me, these are the most important issues when choosing which operation is right for you. For more comprehensive discussion about each procedure, including risks, benefits, and alternatives go to **cliftonthomasmd.com**. Click on Education, log in, and review the different procedures.

All three operations are done laparoscopically. Band patients go home the afternoon of surgery. Bypass and sleeve patients spend one to two days in the hospital. With all three operations, most patients are performing usual activities and back to work within one week.

The diagrams on the following three pages give a visual overview of each surgery.

Skinny Jeans....At Last

Adjustable Gastric Banding

- Laparoscopic
- Least invasive
- Restrictive
- Second-most frequently performed bariatric procedure1
- Mean excess weight loss of 48%
- Requires implanted medical device
- Ongoing maintenance required
- Adjustments/Fills

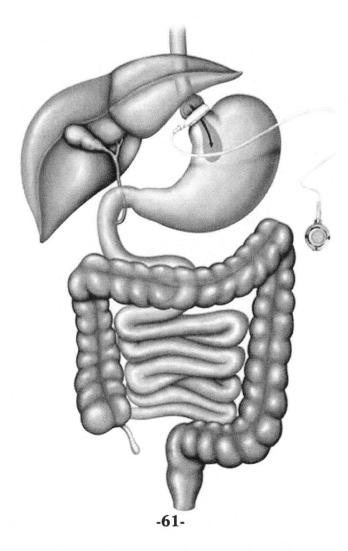

Vertical Sleeve Gastrectomy

- Laparoscopic
- Restrictive
- Mean excess weight loss of 61%
- No implanted medical device

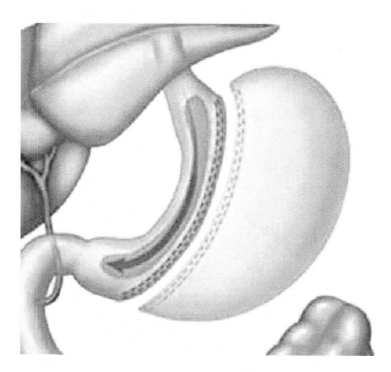

Roux-en-Y Gastric Bypass

- Laparoscopic
- Restrictive/Malabsorptive
- Most frequently performed bariatric procedure
- Mean excess weight loss at 1 year of 62%
- No implanted medical device

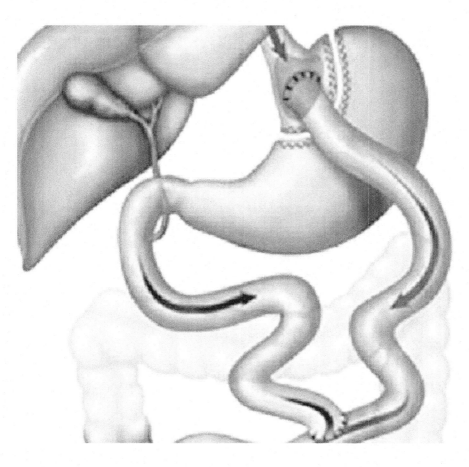

Skinny Jeans....At Last

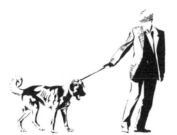

10
WHICH SURGEON IS BEST FOR ME

It happened. Finally, something drove that inner voice inside your head to say, *I want to pursue weight loss surgery*! Now what?

That chatter inside your head is most probably filled with the voices of your closest friends, relatives, or co-workers and their opinions about weight loss surgery (including all the horror stories you or others have heard). Maybe you are remembering images of someone that has been successful. Perhaps you're worried about the cost. Then, you add in those voices that keep asking: *Why can't I do this on my own? What's wrong with me*? For most it is an extremely emotional time.

So I say quiet those voices and think back to the specific *thing* that finally drove you to consider weight loss surgery. Put your energy here. Your amygdala will get busy and help you find the way. Think back to the chapter on what it is like to *fit into those skinny jeans* and remember what drove those people to finally seek a tool like weight loss surgery.

Quiet those voices working against your goal of losing the excess weight and focus on what it is like to fit into those skinny jeans. As you learn, tap into what feels right.

It's time to learn about weight loss surgery and find the best surgeon for you. It's a really big step to finally call and make an appointment. Most likely you are filled with all types of emotions. Remember the book *The Paradox of Choice.* Reduce the anxiety of choosing by having a clear picture of your goal, and avoid making a decision based on emotion.

It may seem like there is a thin line between making an emotional decision and tapping into what feels right, but they are very different.

But what's right for you?

Consider car buying - if you travel or spend much time in your car you may need good gas mileage or instead you may need to choose more on comfort.

I do not want to equate picking a surgeon with buying a car. I just want to make the point of being clear on your goal and tap into what feels right.

Surgeons come in all kinds of different personalities, shapes, and sizes.

So how do you choose the surgeon that is right for you?

First, I want you to have the mindset necessary to make the right choice, and then I will give you a checklist to begin your search.

I am proud to say that, for the most part, bariatric surgery has attracted the best of the best. So, there are many good choices. Most of us who have been doing this for years have a passion for what we do. And it is easy to see why. We get to see the amazing change that occurs as patients reach their goal of fitting into those skinny jeans.

If by chance your surgeon does not seem to have a passion for bariatrics, then look elsewhere. The medical field often likes to depersonalize the physician and surgeon. People do not like this. They like to personalize their choice and choose their surgeon.

We occasionally have a program at our support group meetings called *Profiles of Success*. Patients come and talk about their journey to success. Many say something like, "This is the best money I ever spent, so if you have to beg, borrow, or steal, get it done!" We don't want anyone to steal, but you get the point.

On my website, www.cliftonthomasmd.com there is an affordability calculator. It points out that you save money by having weight loss surgery, often enough to pay cash for it and have that money returned in savings within one to two years.

Enough about the mindset, here is a checklist to begin your search:

☐ Is the surgeon a member of the American Society for Metabolic and Bariatric Surgery?

I am very proud of this organization and have had the pleasure of seeing it grow. It has done an outstanding job of providing the tools we need for excellence and has been responsible for encouraging the development of studies that prove beyond a reasonable doubt we are doing the right thing. It also lets you know that your surgeon is board certified and has the proper credentials.

☐ Is your surgeon a Center of Excellence designee by the Surgical Review Corporation?

Around the year 2000, lots of surgeons suddenly decided to become bariatric surgeons, some with adequate training and some without. Some were prepared and some were not. And there were some very bad outcomes.

Some hospitals were prepared for bariatric patients and some were not. Do you remember the "Good Housekeeping seal of approval?" It was something in the past that put its seal on things of high quality. The SRC is that seal for bariatrics. It requires documentation of all surgeries, complications, volume of surgery, and results in terms of follow up and resolution of medical co-morbidities.

They require low complications and an adequate volume of surgery, as well as documentation of good outcome data on resolution of medical problems. They also require the majority of each surgeaon's practice to be bariatrics. Insurance companies have developed their own brand of "Center of Excellence." I have had an executive from a major insurance company say that the designation has the most to do with marketing and lowest cost. So be careful with the language from the insurance companies.

☐ Does your surgeon have a comprehensive approach with a team of dietitians, counselors, and knowledgeable nurses to guide you through the process?

☐ What hospitals does your surgeon use? And are they designated by the Surgical Review Corporation as a Center of Excellence?

For more info, visit www.surgicalreview.org

☐ What types of weight loss surgeries does your surgeon offer?

Ask the question and watch how the surgeon answers. It will tell you a lot. I personally feel that no one operation fits for all patients. If your surgeon has not done many gastric bypasses, it may be that he is not technically capable.

☐ Does the office staff seem personable?

In the best situations, the office staff reflects the attitude and personality of the surgeon, but often that is not true. So be careful, when judging a surgeon by his office staff. Also, keep in mind that they too are instrumental in your success, so you need to feel comfortable with them.
Remember that bariatric surgery has attracted the best of the best. So if you do not get that feel, look elsewhere.

☐ Do you get a sense that the office billing person will help guide you through the complexity of medical billing and insurance? And will they be responsive to any issues?

Most people do not realize how complicated medical billing is. There are many areas where an issue might arise, so it is important that you get a feel that, they will be responsive.

☐ How well does your surgeon answer your questions?
Pay close attention here.

☐ How well does the office staff answer your questions?

☐ Is the practice website a helpful resource? Is there anything that separates it from the pack?

Let the journey begin. Good luck!

Skinny Jeans....At Last

ABOUT THE AUTHOR

Cliff Thomas' life in the medical field began early. His father was a hospital administrator, and his uncle was a Chief of Staff and primary physician, so essentially he grew up in a hospital. At age 10 he began working in the maintenance department, which evolved into many different jobs around the hospital.

At an early age, Cliff recognized the passion his uncle had for being a doctor. He witnessed it over and over and noticed how his patients responded. That is when the seed was planted. As the years went on, jobs ranged from janitorial to X-ray, to laboratory and finally, to surgery. Cliff realized the best job in the hospital was that of the surgeons'.

He graduated from the University of Texas at Austin in 1979, finishing medical school at the University of Texas Medical Branch in 1984. He then went on to complete a five year General Surgery residency and subsequently became an Assistant Professor of Surgery.

His emphasis throughout residency was GI surgery and included extensive experience with the Vertical Banded Gastroplasty for weight loss, a procedure that was later found to have a 70% failure rate.

Cliff then began a hand surgery fellowship, but it wasn't long before he realized his real passion was GI surgery. He began his solo general surgery practice in Nacogdoches, Texas in 1990, where he continues to have a satellite office today. He chose Nacogdoches because, after his experiences with hand surgery in Oakland, California, he decided smaller was better.

Cliff became a fellow in the American College of Surgeons (FACS) and was Board Certified by the American Board of Surgery in 1990. This year also marked the beginning of laparoscopic surgery, and he quickly found that his skill set fit laparoscopic GI surgery. His advanced laparoscopic experience began in 1992, performing hiatal hernia repairs (Nissen Fundoplications).

At that time there were only a handful of surgeons in the world performing this procedure. It continues to be a rewarding part of his practice and shares many similarities with bariatric surgery.

By the late 1990s, laparoscopic gastric bypass was being performed by several surgeons in the United States. Cliff launched his bariatric surgery practice in 2000, after training with some of the most experienced surgeons in the country and doing a mini-fellowship at Parkland in Dallas.

Since then bariatric surgery has become a major part of his practice. In November 2002 he began also performing the laparoscopic adjustable gastric band and later added the laparoscopic sleeve gastrectomy.

It became clear that Nacogdoches could not support an active bariatric practice, so in 2005 Cliff began practicing in Houston. At that time, Dr. Yusem Nowzaradan and Cliff Thomas performed the largest gastric bypass and gastric sleeve in the world.

Cliff has a passion for what he does, and wakes every morning eager to do more. He gets to use his skill set in surgery, and then see and feel how that changes people's lives for the better.

ADDENDUM

The information on the following pages has been included to give you an extra source of information to help you succeed in your goal of long-term weight loss success.

This addendum includes:

- Supplements Required Following Weight Loss Surgery
- Eating Rules Scoring System
- Obesity -Related Peptides
- The BMI Calculation
- What Does Obesity Look Like?
- Prevalence of Significant Morbidities Per Weight
- Resolution of Morbidities Per Weight Following Surgery
- Bariatric Surgery Low Incidence of Mortality Chart

Skinny Jeans....At Last

SUPPLEMENTS REQUIRED
Following Weight Loss Surgery

These are vitamins that almost every person should take daily whether they have had weight loss surgery or not.

Protein

A person needs a minimum of 50 grams per day. Consider whey protein, the protein in milk, if not eating adequate protein in your meals.

Calcium

1200 to 1500 milligrams per day. Generally 3 tablets of calcium citrate

Vitamin B12

One dissolving tablet under the tongue daily (sublingual)

Vitamin D

Start with 2,000 units per day

Multivitamin

Preferably chewable or liquid. One or two daily. Get a multivitamin with the following included : iron, vitamin A, zinc, and thiamine.

Skinny Jeans....At Last

SUCCESS HABITS SCORING SYSTEM

Score from 10 to 0.

10 = always ; 5 = half the time; 0 = never

_____Plan your meals and follow your plan

_____Go no more than four hours without eating a planned something

_____No unplanned eating (snacking)

_____Drink only liquids with no calories built in

_____Take supplements: calcium, vitamin D, B12, and a multivitamin

Score from 5 to 0.

5 = always; 4/3/2 = sometimes; 0 = never

_____Eat slowly

_____Learning to feel what fullness feels like, not over fullness

_____Do not drink anything while eating a meal

_____Getting comfortable with wasting food

_____Making a daily effort to establish an exercise habit

Score 5 to 0.

5 = never; 4/3/2 = some days; 0 = daily

_____Show love through food with unhealthy food

_____Emotional eating

_____Grazing

_____Skipping meals

_____Drinking carbonated beverages, diet or otherwise

_____ = Total   100

How much weight you lose and your long-term success will follow your success with the above rules. If your score is not perfect, then keep chipping away at it and celebrate your success as you go. Learn to find tools that help you follow these rules.

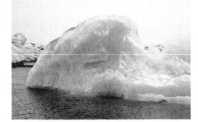

OBESITY RELATED PEPTIDES

Please understand these are just the tip of the iceberg, and more yet-to-be discovered chemicals lie under the surface of what we know.
                              -Clifton Thomas, MD

The following information is complex and this complexity is the essence of why losing weight is so difficult. I suggest looking over the information enough to get the sense that there is more at play with weight regulation than mental weakness.

Obesity results from a massive expansion of white adipose tissue and the recruitment of adipocyte precursor cells. It is a common cause of insulin resistance and diabetes. Increasing evidence suggests that adipose tissue plays an important role in regulating metabolic processes. A complex network of metabolic factors, which include peptide hormones and neurotransmitters, controls these processes. The body produces hormones that act through the brain to regulate short- and long-term appetite, as well as the body's metabolism.

The recent explosion in obesity research has resurrected many peptides whose functions were either unknown, poorly understood or associated with other bioprocesses not believed to be tied to energy homeostasis. In addition, the reverse pharmacology approach utilizing peptide libraries has been instrumental in identifying new endogenous ligands for the vast array of orphan receptors, many of which have been implicated in obesity.

Many different hormones control our weight and appetite. The discovery of new peptide hormones, which suppresses appetite for up to twelve hours, may lead to a better understanding of this complex control system. Hormones that control eating, such as leptin and insulin, circulate in the blood at concentrations proportional to body-fat mass. They decrease appetite by inhibiting neurons that produce the molecules NPY and AGRP, while stimulating melanocortin-producing neurons in the arcuate-nucleus region of the hypothalamus, near the third ventricle of the brain. NPY and AGRP stimulate eating, and melanocortins inhibit eating, via other neurons. Activation of NPY/AGRP-expressing neurons inhibits melanocortin-producing neurons. The gastric hormone ghrelin stimulates appetite by activating the NPY/AGRP-expressing neurons. Batterham and co-workers have shown that PYY (3-36), released from the colon, inhibits these neurons and thereby decreases appetite for up to twelve hours. PYY (3-36) works in part through the auto-inhibitory NPY receptor Y2R.

Central Command Centers

The arcuate nucleus (ARC) of the brain contains two sets of neurons with opposing effects. Activation of the AGRP/NPY neurons increases appetite and metabolism, whereas activation of the POMC/CART neurons has the opposite effect. These neurons connect with second-order neurons in other brain centers, and from there the signals are transmitted through the nucleus tratus solitarius (NTS) to the body. Many appetite-regulating hormones work through the ARC, although they may have direct effects on the NTS and other brain centers as well.

The Peptides

Adiponectin
Adrenomedullin (ADM)
Agouti-Related Protein (AGRP)
Beacon

Bombesin

Bombinakinin-GAP

CART

CCK

Calcitonin Receptor-Stimulating Peptide (CRSP)

Corticotropin Releasing Factor (CRF)

Dynorphin

β-Endorphin

Galanin

Galanin-like peptide (GALP)

Ghrelin

Growth hormone releasing factor (GHRF)

Glucagon-like Peptide-1 (GLP-1)

Gastrin-releasing peptide (GRP)

High Mobility Group Protein Isoform I-C (HMGIC)

HS014

IInsulin

JKC363

Leptin

Melanin Concentrating Hormone (MCH)

Melanocyte Stimulating Hormone (MSH)

Melatonan 2 (MT-2)

Neuromedin

Neurotensin

NPW/NPB

Neuropeptide Y (NPY)

Orexin A/B

Oxytocin

Pituitary Adenylate Cyclase-Activating Polypeptide (PACAP)

Proopiomelanocortin (POMC)

Peptide YY3-36 (PYY 3-36)

Resistin

Secretin

Somatostatin

Skinny Jeans....At Last

TIP39
Thyrotropin Releasing Hormone (TRH)
Uncoupling Protein 3 (UCP3)
Urocortin

THE BMI CALCULATION

What is Morbid Obesity?

- Multifactorial disease of excess fat storage with a genetic basis
- Associated with multiple serious medical problems
- Influenced by the environment
- Lifelong and progressive

$$BMI = \frac{weight\ (kg)}{height\ (m)^2}$$

or

$$BMI = \frac{weight\ (lb)* 703}{height\ (in)^2}$$

- An objective measure of obesity
- Central vs. peripheral obesity

Various Levels of BMI

Normal 18.5 - 24.9

Overweight 25 - 29.9

Obese 30+

      Class 1 30 - 34.9

      Class 2 35 - 39.9

      Class 3 40+

Morbid Obesity more than 100 pounds overweight or a BMI of 40+

What Does Morbid Obesity Look Like?

Normal Weight
(BMI 19 to 24.9)

Overweight
(BMI 25 to 29.9)

Obese (Class I)
(BMI 30 to 34.9)

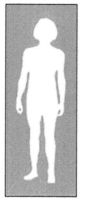
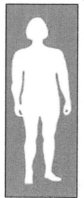
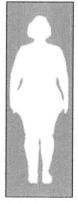

130#
BMI 22

152#
BMI 26

175#
BMI 30

Obese (Class II)
(BMI 35 to 39.9)

Morbidly Obese
(BMI 40 or more)

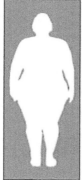
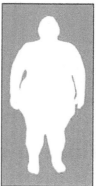

205#
BMI 35

234#
BMI 40

Prevalence of Significant Morbidities per Weight

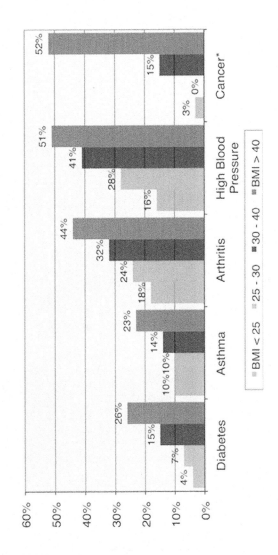

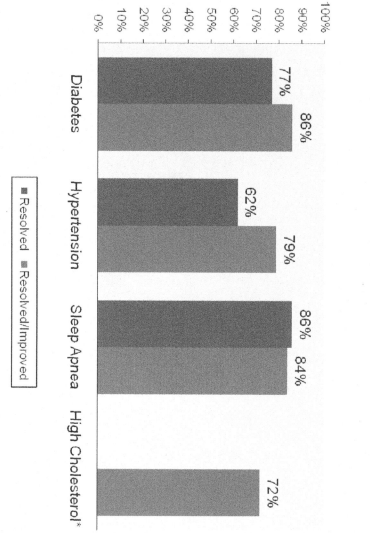

Resolution* of Co-morbidities Following Gastric Bypass Surgery

- Resolved
- Resolved/Improved

Diabetes: 77%, 86%

Hypertension: 62%, 79%

Sleep Apnea: 86%, 84%

High Cholesterol*: 72%

Bariatric Surgery Has a Low Incidence of Mortality

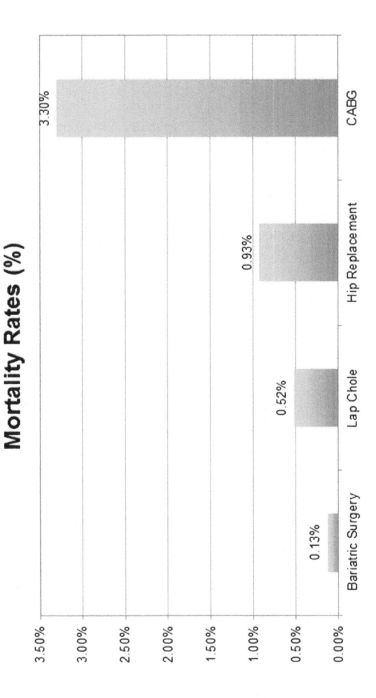

Mortality Rates (%)

REFERENCES

PAGE 83

Agency for Healthcare Research and Quality. Screening for obesity in adults. Accessed June 22, 2010 from http://www.ahrq.gov/clinic/3rdusp-stf/obesity/obeswh.htm

PAGE 84

Agency for Healthcare Research and Quality. Screening for obesity in adults. Accessed June 22, 2010 from http://www.ahrq.gov/clinic/3rdusp-stf/obesity/obeswh.htm
Dugdale DC. Obesity. MedlinePlus. Accessed June 22, 2010 from http://www.nlm.nih.gov/medlineplus/ency/article/007297.htm

PAGE 85

Mokdad AH, Ford ES, Bowman BA, et al. Prevalence of obesity, diabetes, and obesity-related health risk factors, 2001. JAMA 2003;289:76."
* Increase in mortality rate from cancers of all kinds compared to lowest risk group (BMI 25-30). From Calle EE, Rodriguez C, Walker-Thurmond K,et al. Overweight, obesity and mortality from cancer in a prospectively studies cohort of US adults. New Engl J Med 2003;348:1625."

PAGE 86

Buchwald H, Avidor Y, Braunwald E, et al. Bariatric Surgery–A Systematic Review of the Literature and Meta-analysis. JAMA 2004 Oct 13;292(14).

References continued

PAGE 87

1Mortality rate when performed at a Bariatric Surgery Center of Excellence; Bariatric Surgery: DeMaria EJ, Pate V, Warthen M et al. Baseline data from American Society for Metabolic and Bariatric Surgery-designated Bariatric Surgery Centers of Excellence using the Bariatric Outcomes Longitudinal Database, Surgery for Obesity and Related Diseases. Article in Press.

2Dolan JP, Diggs BS, Sheppard BC et al. The National Mortality Burden and Significant Factors Associated with Open and Laparoscopic Cholecystectomy: 1997–2006. J Gastrointest Surg. 2009. Lie SA, Engesaeter LB, Havelin LI et al. Early postoperative mortality after 67,548 total hip replacements. Acta Orthopaedica 2002. Ricciardi R; Virnig BA, Ogilvie Jr. JW. Volume-Outcome Relationship for Coronary Artery Bypass Grafting in an Era of Decreasing Volume. Arch Surg. 2008.

Made in the USA
Monee, IL
06 January 2022

88267166R00056